The Complete Zero Point Recipes for Weight Loss

A Comprehensive Guide to Flavorful, Nutrient-Rich Recipes Designed to Ignite Your Weight Loss Journey and Enhance Your Overall Wellbeing.

DR. HELENA M. OLIVIA

Copyright Page

TABLE OF CONTENTS

Concept of Zero Point Foods 4

Benefits of Zero Point Foods for Weight Loss 6

Stuffed Portobello Mushrooms 8

Tomato Gazpacho 10

Cucumber Gazpacho 12

Broccoli Slaw with Apple Cider Vinegar Dressing 14

Grilled Chicken Caesar Salad 16

Spicy Grilled Shrimp Skewers 18

Steamed Sugar Snap Peas with Sesame Seeds 20

Turkey and Veggie Wrap 22

Roaster Garlic Mushrooms 24

Smoked Salmon Cucumber Bites 26

Celery Sticks with Peanut Butter 28

Sliced Jicama with Lime Juice and Chili Powder 30

Steamed Asparagus with Lemon Juice 32

Cabbage Slaw with Apple Cider

Vinegar Dressing 34

Vegetarian Stir-Fry 36

Roasted Bell Pepper Strips with Hummus 38

Steamed Edamame Beans 40

Roasted Edamame Beans 42

Sauteed Spinach with Garlic and

Red Pepper Flakes 44

Shrimp and Zucchini Noodles 48

Sliced Cucumber with Tzatziki Sauce   50

Grilled Fish Tacos   52

Buffalo Chicken Lettuce Wraps   54

Veggie Omelette   56

Sliced Apples with Cinnamon   58

Greek Chicken Pita Pocket   60

Mango Shrimp Salad   66

Sesame Snap Peas   68

Mushroom and Spinach Quesadilla   70

30-Day Meal Plan   74

Zero Point Food List   76

Important Notice   80

CONCEPT OF ZERO POINT FOODS

Zero Point Foods are foods that have a low or zero SmartPoints value in certain diet programs. These programs assign points to different foods based on their nutritional content. The idea behind Zero Point Foods is that you can enjoy these foods without having to count their points towards your daily allowance. The specific Zero Point Foods can vary depending on the diet program you're following. Usually, these foods are low in calories and high in nutrients, like fruits, vegetables, lean proteins, and whole grains. Since they are lower in calories, you can eat them in larger quantities without worrying about going over your daily points. Including Zero Point Foods in your meals and snacks can help you feel satisfied while staying on track with your goals. They provide a great opportunity to make healthier choices and incorporate more nutritious options into your diet.

- **Weight Loss Programs:** Zero point foods are commonly featured in weight loss programs that utilize a points-based system to help individuals track their food intake. These programs assign points to different foods based on their nutritional content, with the goal of encouraging healthier eating habits and portion control.

- **Zero Point Value:** Foods designated as zero point foods are given a point value of zero, meaning individuals can consume them without counting them towards their daily point allowance. This encourages the consumption of these foods as part of a balanced diet.

- **Nutrient Density:** Zero point foods are typically nutrient-dense, meaning they provide a high amount of nutrients relative to their calorie content. These foods often include fruits, vegetables, lean proteins, and certain whole grains. By focusing on these foods, individuals can increase their intake of essential vitamins, minerals, and fiber while keeping their calorie intake in check.

- **Portion Control:** While zero point foods may be assigned zero points, portion control is still important. Consuming excessive amounts of these foods can still contribute to weight gain. Weight loss programs often provide guidance on portion sizes to help individuals make informed choices about their food intake.

- **Flexibility:** Zero point foods offer flexibility within the program, allowing individuals to build meals and snacks around these foods without feeling restricted. This flexibility can help individuals adhere to their dietary goals over the long term and maintain a balanced and sustainable approach to eating.

BENEFITS OF ZERO POINT FOODS FOR WEIGHT LOSS

- **Low in Calories:** Zero point foods are typically low in calories, which means you can consume them in larger quantities without significantly increasing your overall calorie intake. This can help you feel satisfied and full while still adhering to a calorie deficit, which is necessary for weight loss.

- **High in Nutrients:** Despite being low in calories, zero point foods are often rich in essential nutrients such as vitamins, minerals, and antioxidants. Consuming a variety of nutrient-dense foods supports overall health and well-being, ensuring you get the necessary nutrients while cutting calories for weight loss.

- **Promotes Satiety:** Many zero point foods are high in fiber, water, and protein, all of which contribute to feelings of fullness and satiety. By incorporating these foods into your meals, you can help control hunger and cravings, making it easier to stick to your weight loss plan without feeling deprived.

- **Encourages Healthy Eating Habits:** By focusing on these foods, you naturally reduce your intake of less healthy options like processed foods, sugary snacks, and high-fat foods, promoting a healthier overall diet.

- **Flexibility and Variety:** Zero point foods offer flexibility in meal planning and allow for a wide variety of food choices. This can help prevent boredom with your diet and make it easier to stick to your weight loss goals in the long term.

- **Supports Sustainable Weight Loss:** Because zero point foods are nutritious, filling, and satisfying, they support sustainable weight loss by providing a foundation for a balanced and enjoyable eating plan.

- **Blood Sugar Control:** Foods like non-starchy vegetables and lean proteins have minimal impact on blood sugar levels, which is beneficial for individuals with diabetes or those looking to stabilize their blood sugar levels.

STUFFED PORTOBELLO MUSHROOMS

 Prep Time
20 Mins

Cook Time
25 Mins

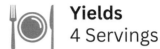 **Yields**
4 Servings

INGREDIENTS

- 2 large bell peppers (any color), sliced
- 2 ripe avocados
- 1 small tomato, diced
- 1/4 cup red onion, finely chopped
- 1 clove garlic, minced
- Juice of 1 lime
- Salt and pepper to taste
- Optional: chopped cilantro for garnish

DIRECTIONS

- In a medium-sized bowl, scoop out the avocados and mash them with a fork until smooth.
- Add diced tomato, chopped red onion, minced garlic, lime juice, salt, and pepper to the mashed avocado. Mix until well combined.
- Taste and adjust seasoning if necessary.
- Arrange the sliced bell peppers on a serving platter.
- Serve the guacamole alongside the sliced bell peppers.
- Garnish with chopped cilantro if desired.
- Enjoy your Zero Point Sliced Bell Peppers with Guacamole!

NUTRITIONAL FACTS
(PER SERVING)

- Calories: 170kcal
- Total Fat: 12g
- Saturated Fat: 1.5g
- Cholesterol: 0mg
- Sodium: 10mg
- Carbohydrates: 16g
- Dietary Fiber: 9g
- Sugars: 4g
- Protein: 3g

TOMATO GAZPACHO

 Prep Time
15 Mins

Cook Time
0 Mins

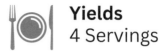 **Yields**
4 Servings

INGREDIENTS

- 6 medium ripe tomatoes, chopped
- 1 cucumber, peeled and chopped
- 1 red bell pepper, chopped
- 1 small red onion, chopped
- 2 cloves garlic, minced
- 2 tablespoons red wine vinegar
- 2 tablespoons olive oil
- Salt and pepper to taste
- 2 cups vegetable broth
- Fresh basil leaves for garnish (optional)

DIRECTIONS

- In a blender, combine tomatoes, cucumber, bell pepper, onion, garlic, red wine vinegar, olive oil, salt, and pepper. Blend until smooth.
- Add vegetable broth to achieve desired consistency. Blend again until well combined.
- Taste and adjust seasoning if necessary.
- Refrigerate for at least 2 hours before serving to allow flavors to meld.
- Serve chilled, garnished with fresh basil leaves if desired.

NUTRITIONAL FACTS (PER SERVING)

- Calories: 80kcal
- Total Fat: 4g
- Saturated Fat: 0.5g
- Cholesterol: 0mg
- Sodium: 320mg
- Carbohydrates: 11g
- Dietary Fiber: 3g
- Sugars: 6g
- Protein: 2g

CUCUMBER GAZPACHO

 Prep Time
15 Mins

Cook Time
0 Mins

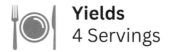 **Yields**
4 Servings

INGREDIENTS

- 3 large cucumbers, peeled and chopped
- 1 green bell pepper, chopped
- 1/2 red onion, chopped
- 2 cloves garlic, minced
- 2 tablespoons red wine vinegar
- 1 tablespoon lemon juice
- Salt and pepper to taste
- 1 cup low-fat Greek yogurt
- 1/4 cup fresh dill, chopped
- 1/4 cup fresh parsley, chopped
- 2 cups vegetable broth

DIRECTIONS

- In a blender, combine cucumbers, bell pepper, onion, garlic, red wine vinegar, lemon juice, salt, and pepper. Blend until smooth.
- Add Greek yogurt, dill, and parsley. Blend again until well combined.
- Gradually add vegetable broth until desired consistency is reached. Blend until smooth.
- Taste and adjust seasoning if necessary.
- Refrigerate for at least 2 hours before serving to allow flavors to meld.
- Serve chilled, garnished with additional fresh herbs if desired.

NUTRITIONAL FACTS (PER SERVING)

- Calories: 70kcal
- Total Fat: 1.5g
- Saturated Fat: 0.5g
- Cholesterol: 5mg
- Sodium: 410mg
- Carbohydrates: 10g
- Dietary Fiber: 2g
- Sugars: 6g
- Protein: 6g

BROCCOLI SLAW WITH APPLE CIDER VINEGAR DRESSING

 Prep Time
10 Mins

Cook Time
0 Mins

 Yields
4 Servings

INGREDIENTS

For the Broccoli Slaw:
- 1 (12 oz) bag of broccoli slaw mix
- 1/2 cup red onion, finely chopped
- 1/2 cup carrots, shredded
- 1/4 cup fresh parsley, chopped

For the Dressing:
- 1/4 cup apple cider vinegar
- 2 tablespoons lemon juice
- 2 teaspoons Dijon mustard
- 1 teaspoon honey (optional, or substitute with your preferred sweetener)
- Salt and pepper to taste.

DIRECTIONS

- In a large mixing bowl, combine the broccoli slaw mix, chopped red onion, shredded carrots, and chopped parsley. Toss well to combine.
- In a small bowl, whisk together the apple cider vinegar, lemon juice, Dijon mustard, honey (if using), salt, and pepper until well combined.
- Pour the dressing over the broccoli slaw mixture. Toss until the slaw is evenly coated with the dressing.

NUTRITIONAL FACTS (PER SERVING)

- Calories: 40kcal
- Total Fat: 0g
- Saturated Fat: 0g
- Cholesterol: 0mg
- Carbohydrates: 10g
- Dietary Fiber: 3g
- Sugars: 4g
- Protein: 2g

DIRECTIONS

- Cover the bowl with plastic wrap or transfer the slaw to an airtight container. Chill in the refrigerator for at least 30 minutes before serving to allow the flavors to meld together.

GRILLED CHICKEN CAESAR SALAD

 Prep Time
10 Mins

Cook Time
15 Mins

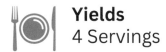 **Yields**
4 Servings

INGREDIENTS

- 4 boneless, skinless chicken breasts
- Salt and pepper, to taste
- 1 tablespoon olive oil
- 1 head romaine lettuce, washed and chopped
- 1/4 cup grated Parmesan cheese
- Caesar salad dressing (use a low-fat or homemade version for fewer points)
- Optional: Croutons (consider using whole grain for fewer points)

DIRECTIONS

- Preheat grill to medium-high heat.
- Season chicken breasts with salt, pepper, and olive oil.
- Grill chicken for about 6-7 minutes per side, or until cooked through (internal temperature of 165°F or 75°C).
- Remove chicken from grill and let it rest for a few minutes before slicing.

Salad Assembly:

- In a large bowl, toss chopped romaine lettuce with grated Parmesan cheese.
- Divide the lettuce among 4 plates.
- Top each plate with sliced grilled chicken.

NUTRITIONAL FACTS (PER SERVING)

- Calories: 180kcal
- Protein: 30g
- Fat: 5g
- Carbohydrates: 3g
- Fiber: 2g

DIRECTIONS

- Drizzle Caesar dressing over the salads according to your preference.
- If desired, sprinkle with croutons.

SPICY GRILLED SHRIMP SKEWERS

 Prep Time
20 Mins

Cook Time
8 Mins

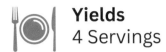 **Yields**
4 Servings

INGREDIENTS

- 1 lb large shrimp, peeled and deveined
- 2 cloves garlic, minced
- 1 tablespoon olive oil
- 1 teaspoon paprika
- 1/2 teaspoon cayenne pepper (adjust according to your spice preference)
- 1/2 teaspoon black pepper
- 1/2 teaspoon salt
- 1 tablespoon fresh parsley, chopped (for garnish)
- Lemon wedges (for serving)

DIRECTIONS

- If you're using wooden skewers, soak them in water for about 30 minutes to prevent burning.
- In a bowl, mix together minced garlic, olive oil, paprika, cayenne pepper, black pepper, and salt.
- Add the shrimp to the bowl and toss until they are evenly coated with the spice mixture. Allow the shrimp to marinate for at least 15 minutes.
- Preheat your grill to medium-high heat.
- Thread the shrimp onto the skewers, distributing them evenly.

NUTRITIONAL FACTS (PER SERVING)

- Calories: 150kcal
- Protein: 24g
- Fat: 4g
- Carbohydrates: 2g
- Fiber: 0.5g
- Sodium: 380mg

DIRECTIONS

- Place the skewers on the grill and cook for about 2-3 minutes per side, or until the shrimp are pink and opaque.
- Once cooked, remove the skewers from the grill and garnish with chopped parsley.
- Serve hot with lemon wedges on the side.

STEAMED SUGAR SNAP PEAS WITH SESAME SEEDS

 Prep Time
10 Mins

Cook Time
5 Mins

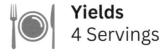 **Yields**
4 Servings

INGREDIENTS

- 1 pound sugar snap peas, trimmed
- 1 tablespoon sesame seeds
- 1 teaspoon soy sauce (optional)
- 1 teaspoon sesame oil (optional)
- Salt, to taste
- Pepper, to taste

DIRECTIONS

- Rinse the sugar snap peas under cold water and pat them dry with a kitchen towel.
- Heat a large pot of water over high heat until it boils. Place a steamer basket over the pot.
- Add the sugar snap peas to the steamer basket, cover, and steam for about 3-5 minutes, or until they are tender-crisp. Be careful not to overcook them.
- While the peas are steaming, heat a small skillet over medium heat. Add the sesame seeds to the skillet and toast them, stirring frequently, until they turn golden brown and fragrant,

NUTRITIONAL FACTS (PER SERVING)

- Calories: 45kcal
- Total Fat: 2g
- Saturated Fat: 0.3g
- Cholesterol: 0mg
- Sodium: 50mg
- Carbohydrates: 5g
- Dietary Fiber: 2g
- Sugars: 2g
- Protein: 2g

DIRECTIONS

- about 2-3 minutes. Remove from heat and set aside.
- Once the sugar snap peas are done steaming, transfer them to a serving dish. If desired, drizzle with soy sauce and sesame oil for added flavor. Season with salt and pepper to taste.
- Sprinkle the toasted sesame seeds over the sugar snap peas and toss gently to coat.
- Serve hot as a side dish or a healthy snack.

TURKEY AND VEGGIE WRAP

 Prep Time
15 Mins

Cook Time
0 Mins

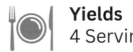 **Yields**
4 Servings

INGREDIENTS

- 4 large lettuce leaves (such as romaine or butter lettuce)
- 8 slices of deli turkey breast
- 1/2 cup shredded carrots
- 1/2 cup shredded cucumber
- 1/2 cup shredded red cabbage
- 1/4 cup sliced bell peppers (any color)
- 1/4 cup sliced red onion
- 4 tablespoons fat-free Greek yogurt
- 2 tablespoons mustard
- Salt and pepper to taste

DIRECTIONS

- Lay out the lettuce leaves on a clean surface.
- In each lettuce leaf, layer 2 slices of turkey breast.
- Divide the shredded carrots, cucumber, red cabbage, bell peppers, and red onion evenly among the lettuce wraps, placing them on top of the turkey slices.
- In a small bowl, mix together the Greek yogurt and mustard. Spread this mixture evenly over the veggies in each wrap.
- Season with salt and pepper to taste.
- Roll up the wraps tightly, tucking in the sides as you go.
- Serve immediately or refrigerate until ready to eat.

22

NUTRITIONAL FACTS
(PER SERVING)

- Calories: 70kcal
- Total Fat: 0.5g
- Saturated Fat: 0g
- Cholesterol: 15mg
- Sodium: 390mg
- Carbohydrates: 5g
- Dietary Fiber: 1.5g
- Sugars: 2g
- Protein: 12g

ROASTED GARLIC MUSHROOMS

 Prep Time
10 Mins

Cook Time
20 Mins

 Yields
4 Servings

INGREDIENTS

- 1 lb (450g) mushrooms (any variety you prefer)
- 4 cloves garlic, minced
- 2 tablespoons fresh parsley, chopped
- Salt and pepper, to taste
- Cooking spray

DIRECTIONS

- Preheat your oven to 400°F (200°C).
- Clean the mushrooms and trim any tough stems. If they are large, you can halve or quarter them.
- In a large bowl, combine the mushrooms, minced garlic, chopped parsley, salt, and pepper. Toss well to coat the mushrooms evenly with the garlic and parsley.
- Lightly coat a baking sheet with cooking spray.
- Spread the seasoned mushrooms out on the baking sheet in a single layer.

NUTRITIONAL FACTS (PER SERVING)

- Calories: 40kcal
- Fat: 1g
- Carbohydrates: 7g
- Protein: 3g
- Fiber: 2g
- Sugar: 2g
- Sodium: 5mg

DIRECTIONS

- Roast in the preheated oven for about 20 minutes, or until the mushrooms are tender and golden brown, stirring once halfway through cooking.
- Once done, remove from the oven and serve hot.

SMOKED SALMON CUCUMBER BITES

 Prep Time
10 Mins

Cook Time
20 Mins

 Yields
20 Pieces

INGREDIENTS

- 1 lb (450g) mushrooms (any variety you prefer)
- 4 cloves garlic, minced
- 2 tablespoons fresh parsley, chopped
- Salt and pepper, to taste
- Cooking spray

DIRECTIONS

- Wash the cucumber thoroughly and pat it dry.
- Cut the cucumber into thin rounds, about 1/4 inch thick. You should get about 20 slices.
- In a small bowl, mix together the fat-free Greek yogurt, chopped dill, capers, lemon zest, salt, and pepper.
- Place the cucumber rounds on a serving platter.
- Spoon a small amount of the yogurt mixture onto each cucumber round.
- Top each cucumber round with a small piece of smoked salmon.
- Garnish the bites with extra dill or a small lemon wedge if desired.

NUTRITIONAL FACTS (PER SERVING)

- **Serving Size:** 1 cucumber bite

- Calories: 20kcal
- Total Fat: 0.5g
- Saturated Fat: 0g
- Cholesterol: 5mg
- Sodium: 65mg
- Carbohydrates: 1g
- Dietary Fiber: 0g
- Sugars: 0g
- Protein: 3g

DIRECTIONS

- Serve immediately or refrigerate until ready to serve.

CELERY STICKS WITH PEANUT BUTTER

 Prep Time
5 Mins

Cook Time
0 Mins

 Yields
4 Servings

INGREDIENTS

- Celery sticks
- Peanut butter (look for low-fat or natural varieties for a healthier option)

DIRECTIONS

- Wash and dry the celery stalks thoroughly.
- Cut the celery stalks into manageable sticks, about 4-5 inches in length.
- Spread peanut butter onto one side of each celery stick.
- Serve immediately, or store in the refrigerator for later consumption.

NUTRITIONAL FACTS (PER SERVING)

- Calories: 100kcal
- Total Fat: 8g
- Saturated Fat: 2g
- Sodium: 100mg
- Carbohydrates: 5g
- Fiber: 2g
- Sugars: 2g
- Protein: 5g

SLICED JICAMA WITH LIME JUICE AND CHILI POWDER

 Prep Time
15 Mins

Cook Time
0 Mins

 Yields
4 Servings

INGREDIENTS

- 1 medium jicama, peeled and sliced into thin rounds or sticks
- Juice of 2 limes
- 1-2 teaspoons chili powder (adjust to taste)
- Salt to taste
- Optional: chopped fresh cilantro for garnish.

DIRECTIONS

- Peel the jicama and slice it into thin rounds or sticks using a sharp knife or a mandoline slicer.
- Place the sliced jicama in a large bowl.
- Squeeze the juice of two limes over the jicama slices.
- Sprinkle chili powder and salt over the jicama.
- Toss well to ensure the jicama slices are evenly coated with lime juice, chili powder, and salt.
- Optional: Garnish with chopped fresh cilantro.
- Serve immediately or refrigerate until ready to serve.

NUTRITIONAL FACTS (PER SERVING)

- Calories: 40kcal
- Total Fat: 0g
- Saturated Fat: 0g
- Cholesterol: 0mg
- Carbohydrates: 10g
- Dietary Fiber: 6g
- Sugars: 2g
- Protein: 1g

STEAMED ASPARAGUS WITH LEMON JUICE

 Prep Time
5 Mins

Cook Time
5 Mins

 Yields
4 Servings

INGREDIENTS

- 1 bunch of fresh asparagus
- 1 lemon
- Salt and pepper to taste

DIRECTIONS

- Preparation: Trim the tough ends off the asparagus spears. You can do this by bending the bottom end of each spear until it snaps naturally. Discard the tough ends.
- Steam Asparagus: Place a steamer basket in a pot filled with about an inch of water. Bring the water to a boil over medium-high heat. Once boiling, add the trimmed asparagus to the steamer basket. Cover the pot and steam for about 3-5 minutes, or until the asparagus is tender yet still crisp.

NUTRITIONAL FACTS (PER SERVING)

- Calories: 20kcal
- Total Fat: 0g
- Saturated Fat: 0g
- Cholesterol: 0mg
- Sodium: 0mg
- Carbohydrates: 5g
- Dietary Fiber: 2g
- Sugars: 1g
- Protein: 2g

DIRECTIONS

- Seasoning: While the asparagus is steaming, zest the lemon and set aside. Once the asparagus is done, transfer it to a serving dish. Squeeze the juice from the lemon over the asparagus and sprinkle with lemon zest, salt, and pepper to taste.
- Serve: Serve the steamed asparagus with lemon juice immediately.

CABBAGE SLAW WITH APPLE CIDER VINEGAR DRESSING

 Prep Time
15 Mins

Cook Time
0 Mins

 Yields
4 Servings

INGREDIENTS

- 4 cups shredded cabbage (green or red)
- 1 cup shredded carrots
- 1 cup shredded apples
- 1/4 cup finely chopped red onion
- 2 tablespoons apple cider vinegar
- 1 tablespoon Dijon mustard
- 1 tablespoon honey or preferred sweetener (optional)
- Salt and pepper to taste
- Fresh parsley or cilantro for garnish (optional)

DIRECTIONS

- In a large mixing bowl, combine the shredded cabbage, carrots, shredded apples, and chopped red onion.
- In a small bowl, whisk together the apple cider vinegar, Dijon mustard, and honey (if using). Adjust sweetness to your preference.
- Pour the dressing over the cabbage mixture and toss until well combined and evenly coated.
- Season with salt and pepper to taste.
- Allow the slaw to sit for at least 10-15 minutes before serving to allow the flavors to meld together.

DIRECTIONS

- Garnish with fresh parsley or cilantro if desired before serving.
- Enjoy your zero-point cabbage slaw with apple cider vinegar dressing as a refreshing side dish or topping for tacos, sandwiches, or wraps!

VEGETARIAN STIR-FRY

 Prep Time
15 Mins

Cook Time
10 Mins

 Yields
4 Servings

INGREDIENTS

- 1 tablespoon olive oil spray
- 2 cloves garlic, minced
- 1 small onion, thinly sliced
- 1 bell pepper, thinly sliced
- 2 cups sliced mushrooms
- 2 cups broccoli florets
- 1 cup snap peas
- 1 cup shredded carrots
- 2 tablespoons low-sodium soy sauce
- 1 tablespoon rice vinegar
- 1 teaspoon sesame oil
- Salt and pepper to taste
- Optional: red pepper flakes for added spice
- Optional toppings: chopped green onions, sesame seeds

DIRECTIONS

- Heat olive oil spray in a large skillet or wok over medium-high heat.
- Add minced garlic and sliced onion to the skillet, sauté for 1-2 minutes until fragrant.
- Add bell pepper, mushrooms, broccoli, snap peas, and shredded carrots to the skillet. Stir-fry for about 5-7 minutes until the vegetables are tender yet crisp.
- In a small bowl, mix together soy sauce, rice vinegar, sesame oil, salt, pepper, and red pepper flakes if using.
- Pour the sauce over the vegetables in the skillet and toss to coat evenly. Cook for an additional 1-2 minutes until heated through.

NUTRITIONAL FACTS (PER SERVING)

- Calories: 100kcal
- Total Fat: 4g
- Carbohydrates: 15g
- Protein: 6g
- Fiber: 5g

DIRECTIONS

- Taste and adjust seasoning if necessary.
- Serve hot, garnished with chopped green onions and sesame seeds if desired.

ROASTED BELL PEPPER STRIPS WITH HUMMUS

 Prep Time
10 Mins

Cook Time
20 Mins

 Yields
4 Servings

INGREDIENTS

- 2 large bell peppers (red, yellow, or orange)
- 1 tablespoon olive oil
- Salt and pepper to taste
- 1 cup hummus (store-bought or homemade)

DIRECTIONS

- Preheat your oven to 425°F (220°C).
- Wash the bell peppers and pat them dry with a paper towel. Cut each pepper in half lengthwise, then remove the seeds and membranes. Slice the peppers into strips about 1-inch wide.
- In a large bowl, toss the pepper strips with olive oil, salt, and pepper until evenly coated.
- Spread the pepper strips in a single layer on a baking sheet lined with parchment paper or aluminum foil.
- Roast the peppers in the preheated oven for about 15-20 minutes, or until they are tender and slightly charred around the edges,

NUTRITIONAL FACTS (PER SERVING)

- Calories: 150kcal
- Total Fat: 10g
- Saturated Fat: 1g
- Cholesterol: 0mg
- Sodium: 300mg
- Carbohydrates: 12g
- Dietary Fiber: 4g
- Sugars: 2g
- Protein: 4g

DIRECTIONS

- stirring once halfway through cooking.
- While the peppers are roasting, prepare the hummus if you're making it from scratch or take it out of the refrigerator if using store-bought.
- Once the peppers are done, remove them from the oven and let them cool slightly.
- Serve the roasted bell pepper strips with hummus for dipping.

STEAMED EDAMAME BEANS

 Prep Time
5 Mins

Cook Time
5 Mins

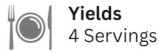 **Yields**
4 Servings

INGREDIENTS

- 2 cups frozen edamame beans (in pods)
- Salt to taste

DIRECTIONS

- Bring a large pot of water to a boil.
- Add frozen edamame beans to the boiling water.
- Cook for about 5 minutes until beans are tender.
- Drain the beans and sprinkle with salt to taste.
- Serve hot or cold.

NUTRITIONAL FACTS (PER SERVING)

- Calories: 100kcal
- Protein: 8g
- Fat: 4g
- Carbohydrates: 8g
- Fiber: 4g

ROASTED EDAMAME BEANS

 Prep Time
5 Mins

Cook Time
20 Mins

 Yields
4 Servings

INGREDIENTS

- 2 cups frozen edamame beans (shelled)
- 1 tablespoon olive oil
- Salt and pepper to taste
- Optional: garlic powder, chili powder, or other seasonings of your choice

DIRECTIONS

- Preheat the oven to 400°F (200°C).
- Pat dry the shelled edamame beans using paper towels to remove excess moisture.
- In a bowl, toss the edamame beans with olive oil, salt, pepper, and any additional seasonings of your choice until evenly coated.
- Spread the seasoned beans in a single layer on a baking sheet.
- Roast in the preheated oven for about 20 minutes, stirring halfway through, until beans are crispy.
- Remove from the oven and let cool slightly before serving.

NUTRITIONAL FACTS (PER SERVING)

- Calories: 120kcal
- Protein: 10g
- Fat: 6g
- Carbohydrates: 8g
- Fiber: 4g

SAUTÉED SPINACH WITH GARLIC AND RED PEPPER FLAKES

 Prep Time
5 Mins

Cook Time
5 Mins

 Yields
4 Servings

INGREDIENTS

- 1 pound fresh spinach leaves, washed and dried
- 3 cloves garlic, minced
- 1/2 teaspoon red pepper flakes (adjust to taste)
- Salt to taste
- 1 tablespoon olive oil (optional)

DIRECTIONS

- Heat olive oil (if using) in a large skillet over medium heat.
- Add minced garlic and red pepper flakes to the skillet. Sauté for about 30 seconds until fragrant, being careful not to burn the garlic.
- Add spinach to the skillet in batches, tossing with tongs until wilted. Continue adding more spinach until it's all in the skillet.
- Cook the spinach for an additional 2-3 minutes, stirring occasionally, until fully wilted and heated through.
- Season with salt to taste.
- Serve hot as a side dish or as a base for other recipes.

NUTRITIONAL FACTS (PER SERVING)

- Calories: 30kcal
- Total Fat: 1g
- Saturated Fat: 0g
- Cholesterol: 0mg
- Sodium: 120mg
- Carbohydrates: 4g
- Dietary Fiber: 2g
- Sugars: 0g
- Protein: 3g

CELERY STICKS WITH PEANUT BUTTER

 Prep Time
5 Mins

Cook Time
0 Mins

 Yields
4 Servings

INGREDIENTS

- Celery sticks
- Peanut butter (look for low-fat or natural varieties for a healthier option)

DIRECTIONS

- Wash and dry the celery stalks thoroughly.
- Cut the celery stalks into manageable sticks, about 4-5 inches in length.
- Spread peanut butter onto one side of each celery stick.
- Serve immediately, or store in the refrigerator for later consumption.

NUTRITIONAL FACTS (PER SERVING)

- Calories: 100kcal
- Total Fat: 8g
- Saturated Fat: 2g
- Sodium: 100mg
- Carbohydrates: 5g
- Fiber: 2g
- Sugars: 2g
- Protein: 5g

SHRIMP AND ZUCCHINI NOODLES

 Prep Time   **Cook Time**
15 Mins   10 Mins

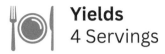 **Yields**
4 Servings

INGREDIENTS

- 1 lb shrimp, peeled and deveined
- 4 medium zucchinis, spiralized
- 2 cloves garlic, minced
- 1 tablespoon olive oil
- Salt and pepper to taste
- Red pepper flakes (optional)
- Fresh parsley for garnish (optional)

DIRECTIONS

- **Prep the Shrimp:** Rinse the shrimp under cold water and pat dry with paper towels. Season with salt and pepper to taste.
- **Prepare Zucchini Noodles:** Spiralize the zucchinis into noodles using a spiralizer. Set aside.
- **Cooking the Shrimp:** Heat olive oil in a large skillet over medium-high heat. Add minced garlic and cook for about 30 seconds until fragrant. Add the shrimp to the skillet and cook for 2-3 minutes on each side until they turn pink and opaque. Remove the shrimp from the skillet and set aside.

NUTRITIONAL FACTS (PER SERVING)

- Calories: 160kcal
- Protein: 25g
- Fat: 4g
- Carbohydrates: 7g
- Fiber: 2g

DIRECTIONS

- **Cooking Zucchini Noodles:** In the same skillet, add the spiralized zucchini noodles. Cook for 2-3 minutes, tossing occasionally, until the noodles are tender but still slightly crisp.
- **Combine:** Once the zucchini noodles are cooked, add the cooked shrimp back to the skillet. Toss everything together until well combined. Adjust seasoning with salt, pepper, and red pepper flakes if desired.
- **Serve:** Divide the shrimp and zucchini noodles among plates. Garnish with fresh parsley if desired.

SLICED CUCUMBER WITH TZATZIKI SAUCE

 Prep Time
15 Mins

Cook Time
10 Mins

 Yields
4 Servings

INGREDIENTS

For Tzatziki Sauce:
- 1 cup Greek yogurt (non-fat for zero points)
- 1 medium cucumber, grated and drained
- 2 cloves garlic, minced
- 1 tablespoon lemon juice
- 1 tablespoon extra virgin olive oil
- 1 tablespoon chopped fresh dill (optional)
- Salt and pepper to taste

For Serving:
- 2 medium cucumbers, sliced
- Fresh dill or mint for garnish (optional)

DIRECTIONS

- **Prepare the Tzatziki Sauce:** In a bowl, combine the Greek yogurt, grated cucumber, minced garlic, lemon juice, olive oil, and chopped dill.
- Mix well until all ingredients are fully incorporated.
- Season with salt and pepper to taste. Adjust seasoning if needed.
- Refrigerate the tzatziki sauce for at least 30 minutes to allow the flavors to meld.
- **Slice the Cucumbers:** Wash and dry the remaining cucumbers.
- Using a sharp knife or a mandoline slicer, thinly slice the cucumbers into rounds.

NUTRITIONAL FACTS (PER SERVING)

- Calories: 40kcal
- Total Fat: 2g
- Saturated Fat: 0g
- Cholesterol: 0mg
- Sodium: 20mg
- Carbohydrates: 3g
- Dietary Fiber: 1g
- Sugars: 2g
- Protein: 3g

DIRECTIONS

- **Assemble:** Arrange the cucumber slices on a serving platter.
- Spoon the prepared tzatziki sauce over the cucumber slices, or serve it on the side as a dipping sauce.
- Garnish with fresh dill or mint leaves, if desired.
- **Serve:** Serve the sliced cucumbers with tzatziki sauce immediately as a refreshing appetizer or snack.

GRILLED FISH TACOS

 Prep Time
10 Mins

Cook Time
8 Mins

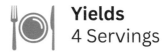 **Yields**
4 Servings

INGREDIENTS

- 1 pound white fish fillets (such as tilapia, cod, or halibut)
- 1 tablespoon olive oil
- 1 teaspoon chili powder
- 1 teaspoon cumin
- 1/2 teaspoon paprika
- Salt and pepper to taste
- 8 small corn tortillas
- Optional toppings: shredded cabbage, sliced avocado, diced tomatoes, cilantro, lime wedges

DIRECTIONS

- **Prepare the Tzatziki Sauce:** In a bowl, combine the Greek yogurt, grated cucumber, minced garlic, lemon juice, olive oil, and chopped dill.
- Mix well until all ingredients are fully incorporated.
- Season with salt and pepper to taste. Adjust seasoning if needed.
- Refrigerate the tzatziki sauce for at least 30 minutes to allow the flavors to meld.
- **Slice the Cucumbers:** Wash and dry the remaining cucumbers.
- Using a sharp knife or a mandoline slicer, thinly slice the cucumbers into rounds.

NUTRITIONAL FACTS (PER SERVING)

- Calories: 150kcal
- Protein: 20g
- Fat: 4g
- Carbohydrates: 10g
- Fiber: 2g
- Sugar: 0g

DIRECTIONS

- **Assemble:** Arrange the cucumber slices on a serving platter.
- Spoon the prepared tzatziki sauce over the cucumber slices, or serve it on the side as a dipping sauce.
- Garnish with fresh dill or mint leaves, if desired.
- **Serve:** Serve the sliced cucumbers with tzatziki sauce immediately as a refreshing appetizer or snack.

BUFFALO CHICKEN LETTUCE WRAPS

 Prep Time
10 Mins

Cook Time
20 Mins

 Yields
4 Servings

INGREDIENTS

- 1 lb boneless, skinless chicken breasts
- 1/2 cup buffalo sauce (choose a low-calorie or sugar-free option for a healthier version)
- 1 teaspoon garlic powder
- Salt and pepper to taste
- Iceberg lettuce leaves, washed and dried.

DIRECTIONS

- Season the chicken breasts with garlic powder, salt, and pepper. Grill or cook them in a skillet over medium heat until they're cooked through. Allow them to cool slightly, then shred the chicken using two forks.
- In a bowl, combine the shredded chicken with buffalo sauce, adjusting the amount to your taste preferences. Mix until the chicken is evenly coated with the sauce.
- Take individual iceberg lettuce leaves and fill each one with a portion of the buffalo chicken mixture.

NUTRITIONAL FACTS (PER SERVING)

- Calories: 200kcal
- Protein: 30g
- Carbohydrates: 3g
- Fat: 6g
- Fiber: 1g

DIRECTIONS

- Optionally, sprinkle diced tomatoes, diced celery, shredded carrots, or blue cheese crumbles on top of the buffalo chicken.
- Arrange the lettuce wraps on a serving platter and serve immediately.

VEGGIE OMELETTE

 Prep Time
5 Mins

Cook Time
10 Mins

 Yields
1 Serving

INGREDIENTS

- 3 large eggs
- 1/4 cup diced bell peppers (any color)
- 1/4 cup diced tomatoes
- 1/4 cup diced onions
- 1/4 cup diced mushrooms
- Salt and pepper to taste
- Cooking spray

DIRECTIONS

- In a mixing bowl, beat the eggs until well combined. Season with salt and pepper according to your taste preferences.
- Heat a non-stick skillet over medium heat and coat it with cooking spray.
- Add the diced bell peppers, tomatoes, onions, and mushrooms to the skillet. Sauté for 3-4 minutes or until the vegetables are slightly softened.
- Pour the beaten eggs over the sautéed vegetables in the skillet. Allow the eggs to cook undisturbed for about 2-3 minutes, or until the edges start to set.

NUTRITIONAL FACTS (PER SERVING)

- Calories: 170kcal
- Total Fat: 10g
- Saturated Fat: 3g
- Cholesterol: 465mg
- Sodium: 240mg
- Carbohydrates: 8g
- Dietary Fiber: 2g
- Sugars: 4g
- Protein: 13g

DIRECTIONS

- Gently lift the edges of the omelette with a spatula and tilt the skillet to let the uncooked egg mixture flow to the edges. Continue cooking for another 2-3 minutes or until the omelette is almost set.
- Carefully fold the omelette in half using the spatula. Cook for an additional 1-2 minutes or until the eggs are fully set.
- Transfer the omelette to a plate and serve hot.

SLICED APPLES WITH CINNAMON

 Prep Time
10 Mins

Cook Time
20 Mins

 Yields
4 Servings

INGREDIENTS

- 4 medium-sized apples
- 1 teaspoon ground cinnamon
- Optional: 1 tablespoon lemon juice (to prevent browning)

DIRECTIONS

- Wash the apples thoroughly under running water. Peel the skin if desired, although leaving the skin on adds extra fiber and nutrients. Core the apples and slice them thinly. If you're concerned about the apples browning, you can toss them with a tablespoon of lemon juice.
- Lay the sliced apples on a serving plate or in a bowl, arranging them neatly.
- Evenly sprinkle ground cinnamon over the sliced apples. Adjust the amount to your taste preference.

NUTRITIONAL FACTS (PER SERVING)

- Calories: 60kcal
- Carbohydrates: 16g
- Dietary Fiber: 3g
- Sugars: 11g
- Protein: 0g

DIRECTIONS

- Serve immediately as a healthy snack or dessert. You can also refrigerate any leftovers for later consumption.

GREEK CHICKEN PITA POCKET

 Prep Time
10 Mins

Cook Time
15 Mins

 Yields
4 Servings

INGREDIENTS

- 2 boneless, skinless chicken breasts
- 1 teaspoon olive oil
- 1 teaspoon dried oregano
- 1 teaspoon dried basil
- 1 teaspoon garlic powder
- Salt and pepper to taste
- 4 whole wheat pita pockets
- 1 cup shredded lettuce
- 1 tomato, diced
- 1/2 cucumber, diced
- 1/4 cup red onion, thinly sliced
- 1/4 cup crumbled feta cheese (optional)
- Tzatziki sauce for serving (optional)

DIRECTIONS

- Preheat your grill or grill pan over medium-high heat.
- In a small bowl, mix together olive oil, oregano, basil, garlic powder, salt, and pepper.
- Brush the chicken breasts with the olive oil mixture.
- Grill the chicken breasts for about 6-8 minutes per side or until cooked through and no longer pink in the middle.
- Once cooked, remove the chicken from the grill and let it rest for a few minutes before slicing it thinly.
- While the chicken is resting, warm the pita pockets according to package instructions.

NUTRITIONAL FACTS (PER SERVING)

- Calories: 250kcal
- Total Fat: 5g
- Saturated Fat: 1g
- Cholesterol: 60mg
- Sodium: 300mg
- Carbohydrates: 25g
- Dietary Fiber: 4g
- Sugars: 2g
- Protein: 25g

DIRECTIONS

- Carefully open each pita pocket and stuff them with shredded lettuce, diced tomato, diced cucumber, sliced red onion, and sliced grilled chicken.
- If desired, sprinkle crumbled feta cheese over the top of each pita pocket.
- Serve the pita pockets with tzatziki sauce on the side for dipping, if desired.

CUCUMBER GAZPACHO

 Prep Time
15 Mins

Cook Time
0 Mins

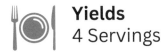 **Yields**
4 Servings

INGREDIENTS

- 3 large cucumbers, peeled and chopped
- 1 green bell pepper, chopped
- 1/2 red onion, chopped
- 2 cloves garlic, minced
- 2 tablespoons red wine vinegar
- 1 tablespoon lemon juice
- Salt and pepper to taste
- 1 cup low-fat Greek yogurt
- 1/4 cup fresh dill, chopped
- 1/4 cup fresh parsley, chopped
- 2 cups vegetable broth

DIRECTIONS

- In a blender, combine cucumbers, bell pepper, onion, garlic, red wine vinegar, lemon juice, salt, and pepper. Blend until smooth.
- Add Greek yogurt, dill, and parsley. Blend again until well combined.
- Gradually add vegetable broth until desired consistency is reached. Blend until smooth.
- Taste and adjust seasoning if necessary.
- Refrigerate for at least 2 hours before serving to allow flavors to meld.
- Serve chilled, garnished with additional fresh herbs if desired.

NUTRITIONAL FACTS
(PER SERVING)

- Calories: 70kcal
- Total Fat: 1.5g
- Saturated Fat: 0.5g
- Cholesterol: 5mg
- Sodium: 410mg
- Carbohydrates: 10g
- Dietary Fiber: 2g
- Sugars: 6g
- Protein: 6g

ROASTED EDAMAME BEANS

 Prep Time
5 Mins

Cook Time
20 Mins

 Yields
4 Servings

INGREDIENTS

- 2 cups frozen edamame beans (shelled)
- 1 tablespoon olive oil
- Salt and pepper to taste
- Optional: garlic powder, chili powder, or other seasonings of your choice

DIRECTIONS

- Preheat the oven to 400°F (200°C).
- Pat dry the shelled edamame beans using paper towels to remove excess moisture.
- In a bowl, toss the edamame beans with olive oil, salt, pepper, and any additional seasonings of your choice until evenly coated.
- Spread the seasoned beans in a single layer on a baking sheet.
- Roast in the preheated oven for about 20 minutes, stirring halfway through, until beans are crispy.
- Remove from the oven and let cool slightly before serving.

NUTRITIONAL FACTS (PER SERVING)

- Calories: 120kcal
- Protein: 10g
- Fat: 6g
- Carbohydrates: 8g
- Fiber: 4g

MANGO SHRIMP SALAD

 Prep Time
15 Mins

Cook Time
0 Mins

 Yields
4 Servings

INGREDIENTS

- 1 lb cooked shrimp, peeled and deveined
- 1 large ripe mango, diced
- 1 red bell pepper, diced
- 1/2 red onion, finely chopped
- 1/4 cup fresh cilantro, chopped
- Juice of 2 limes
- Salt and pepper to taste
- Optional: chili flakes or hot sauce for added heat.

DIRECTIONS

- In a large bowl, combine the cooked shrimp, diced mango, diced red bell pepper, chopped red onion, and chopped cilantro.
- Squeeze the juice of 2 limes over the salad and toss gently to combine.
- Season with salt and pepper to taste. If you like a little heat, add chili flakes or hot sauce to your preference.
- Serve chilled.

NUTRITIONAL FACTS (PER SERVING)

- Calories: 160kcal
- Protein: 20g
- Carbohydrates: 15g
- Fat: 2g
- Fiber: 2g

SESAME SNAP PEAS

 Prep Time
5 Mins

Cook Time
10 Mins

 Yields
4 Servings

INGREDIENTS

- 1 lb snap peas, trimmed
- 2 tablespoons soy sauce (use low-sodium for a healthier option)
- 1 tablespoon rice vinegar
- 1 teaspoon sesame oil
- 1 tablespoon sesame seeds, toasted
- 2 green onions, thinly sliced
- 1 teaspoon minced garlic
- 1 teaspoon minced ginger
- Salt and pepper to taste
- Optional: red pepper flakes for heat.

DIRECTIONS

- Wash and trim the snap peas, removing the stems.
- In a small bowl, mix together soy sauce, rice vinegar, sesame oil, garlic, ginger, and optional red pepper flakes.
- In a large skillet or wok, heat a tablespoon of water over medium-high heat. Add snap peas and stir-fry for about 2-3 minutes until they are crisp-tender.
- Pour the prepared sauce over the snap peas and toss to coat evenly. Cook for an additional 1-2 minutes until the sauce has thickened slightly and coats the snap peas.

NUTRITIONAL FACTS (PER SERVING)

- Calories: 50kcal
- Total Fat: 2g
- Saturated Fat: 0g
- Cholesterol: 0mg
- Sodium: 240mg
- Carbohydrates: 6g
- Dietary Fiber: 2g
- Sugars: 2g
- Protein: 3g

DIRECTIONS

- Transfer the snap peas to a serving dish and sprinkle with toasted sesame seeds and sliced green onions.
- Serve hot as a delicious and healthy side dish.

MUSHROOM AND SPINACH QUESADILLA

 Prep Time
10 Mins

Cook Time
15 Mins

 Yields
2 Servings

INGREDIENTS

- 2 large whole wheat tortillas (approximately 8 inches in diameter)
- 1 cup sliced mushrooms
- 1 cup fresh spinach leaves
- 1/2 cup diced tomatoes
- 1/2 cup diced onions
- 1/2 cup diced bell peppers
- 1/2 cup shredded fat-free mozzarella cheese
- Salt and pepper to taste
- Cooking spray.

DIRECTIONS

- Heat a non-stick skillet over medium heat and coat it with cooking spray.
- Add the mushrooms, onions, and bell peppers to the skillet. Cook until they are softened, about 5-7 minutes.
- Add the spinach leaves to the skillet and cook until wilted, about 2 minutes. Season with salt and pepper to taste.
- Remove the skillet from heat and set aside.
- Wipe the skillet clean and return it to the stove over medium heat.
- Place one tortilla in the skillet and sprinkle half of the cheese evenly over the tortilla.

NUTRITIONAL FACTS (PER SERVING)

- Calories: 200kcal
- Fat: 2g
- Carbohydrates: 30g
- Protein: 10g
- Fiber: 7g

DIRECTIONS

- Spread the cooked mushroom and spinach mixture evenly over the cheese.
- Top with the diced tomatoes and the remaining cheese.
- Place the second tortilla on top and press down gently.
- Cook the quesadilla for 2-3 minutes on each side, or until the tortillas are golden brown and crispy, and the cheese is melted.
- Remove the quesadilla from the skillet and let it cool for a minute before slicing into wedges.
- Serve hot with salsa or your favorite dipping sauce.

MUSHROOM AND SPINACH QUESADILLA

 Prep Time
10 Mins

Cook Time
15 Mins

 Yields
2 Servings

INGREDIENTS

- 2 large whole wheat tortillas (approximately 8 inches in diameter)
- 1 cup sliced mushrooms
- 1 cup fresh spinach leaves
- 1/2 cup diced tomatoes
- 1/2 cup diced onions
- 1/2 cup diced bell peppers
- 1/2 cup shredded fat-free mozzarella cheese
- Salt and pepper to taste
- Cooking spray.

DIRECTIONS

- Heat a non-stick skillet over medium heat and coat it with cooking spray.
- Add the mushrooms, onions, and bell peppers to the skillet. Cook until they are softened, about 5-7 minutes.
- Add the spinach leaves to the skillet and cook until wilted, about 2 minutes. Season with salt and pepper to taste.
- Remove the skillet from heat and set aside.
- Wipe the skillet clean and return it to the stove over medium heat.
- Place one tortilla in the skillet and sprinkle half of the cheese evenly over the tortilla.

NUTRITIONAL FACTS (PER SERVING)

- Calories: 200kcal
- Fat: 2g
- Carbohydrates: 30g
- Protein: 10g
- Fiber: 7g

DIRECTIONS

- Spread the cooked mushroom and spinach mixture evenly over the cheese.
- Top with the diced tomatoes and the remaining cheese.
- Place the second tortilla on top and press down gently.
- Cook the quesadilla for 2-3 minutes on each side, or until the tortillas are golden brown and crispy, and the cheese is melted.
- Remove the quesadilla from the skillet and let it cool for a minute before slicing into wedges.
- Serve hot with salsa or your favorite dipping sauce.

Meal plan

for 30 Days

Date
_____

	BREAKFAST	LUNCH	DINNER
MON	Scrambled eggs with spinach and tomatoes	Grilled chicken breast with a mixed green salad (lettuce, cucumber, bell peppers) and balsamic vinaigrette	Baked salmon with steamed broccoli and cauliflower
TUE	Greek yogurt with fresh berries and a sprinkle of chia seeds	Turkey lettuce wraps with hummus and sliced veggies	Stir-fried shrimp with bell peppers, onions, and zucchini served over cauliflower rice
WED	Oatmeal topped with sliced banana and a dollop of almond butter	Quinoa salad with cherry tomatoes, cucumber, red onion, and lemon-tahini dressing	Grilled tofu with roasted Brussels sprouts and carrots
THU	Veggie omelet (with mushrooms, onions, bell peppers) cooked in olive oil	Lentil soup with a side of mixed greens dressed with lemon juice	Baked cod with asparagus and a side of mixed bean salad
FRI	Smoothie made with spinach, frozen berries, banana, and almond milk	Grilled shrimp skewers with a side of Greek salad (tomatoes, cucumbers, olives, feta cheese)	Zucchini noodles with marinara sauce and grilled chicken breast
SAT	Cottage cheese topped with pineapple chunks and a sprinkle of cinnamon	Tuna salad lettuce wraps with diced celery and carrots	Turkey chili with black beans, diced tomatoes, and bell peppers

Meal plan

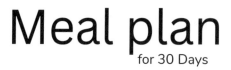

for 30 Days

Date
_____

	BREAKFAST	LUNCH	DINNER
SUN	Whole grain toast with mashed avocado and sliced tomato	Egg salad stuffed in bell pepper halves served with a side of carrot sticks	Grilled steak with roasted green beans and a side of quinoa

Week 2-4

- Continue to repeat and vary these meal ideas throughout the 30-day period, incorporating a wide range of fruits, vegetables, lean proteins, and whole grains. Remember to drink plenty of water throughout the day.

ZERO POINT FOOD LIST

Zero Point Fruits

- Apples
- Apricots
- Bananas
- Blackberries
- Blueberries
- Cantaloupe
- Cherries
- Clementine
- Coconut
- Cranberries
- Dates
- Dragon Fruit
- Figs
- Grapefruit
- Grapes (any variety)
- Guava
- Honeydew Melon
- Jackfruit
- Kiwi
- Lemon
- Lime
- Mango
- Oranges
- Passion Fruit
- Peach
- Pears
- Pineapple

BEANS & LEGUMES

- Adzuki beans
- Alfalfa sprouts
- Bean sprouts
- Black beans
- Black-eyed peas
- Cannellini beans
- Chickpeas
- Edamame
- Fava beans
- Great Northern beans
- Hominy
- Kidney beans
- Lentils
- Lima beans
- Lupini beans
- Navy beans
- Pinto beans
- Refried beans, canned, fat-free
- Soy beans

CHICKEN & TURKEY BREAST

- Ground chicken breast
- Ground turkey, 98% fat-free
- Ground turkey breast
- Skinless chicken breast
- Skinless turkey breast

EGGS

- Egg substitute
- Egg whites
- Egg yolks
- Eggs

Zero Point Vegetables (Starchy & Non-Starchy)

- Arrowroot, raw
- Artichoke
- Arugula
- Asparagus
- Broccoli
- Beans (black, adzuki, cannellini, garbanzo, kidney, great northern, lima, pinto, etc.)
- Beans, refried (canned, fat-free, no added sugar)
- Green Beans
- Bok Choy
- Brussel Sprouts
- Cabbage
- Carrots
- Cauliflower
- Celery
- Chard
- Chickpeas
- Collards
- Corn
- Cucumber
- Daikon
- Edamame
- Eggplant
- Endive
- Fennel
- Ginger Root
- Kale
- Leeks
- Lettuce (any variety)
- Mushrooms
- Okra
- Peas
- Peppers (bell)
- Pickles (without sugar)
- Pumpkin
- Radishes
- Scallions (green onions)
- Spinach
- Sprouts
- Squash
- Tomatoes
- Turnips
- Zucchini

Zero Point Herbs and Spices

- Basil
- Chives
- Cinnamon
- Dill Weed
- Garlic
- Garlic Salt
- Italian Seasoning
- Oregano
- Paprika
- Parsley
- Pepper
- Peppermint
- Pumpkin Spice
- Rosemary
- Sage
- Salt
- Thyme

Zero Point Meat, Seafood and Poultry

- Calamari, grilled
- Chicken Breast (boneless, skinless)
- Crab (Alasaka king, Dungeness, queen, king)
- Crayfish
- Eggs
- Bass Fish
- Bluefish
- Carp
- Catfish
- Cod
- Eel
- Grouper
- Haddock
- Halibut
- Lobster
- Mackerel Fish
- Mussels
- Octopus
- Oysters
- Salmon (Atlantic and farm raised)
- Sardines
- Sea Bass
- Shrimp
- Sturgeon Fish
- Swordfish
- Tilapia Fish

FISH/SHELLFISH

- Abalone
- Alaskan king crab
- Anchovies, in water
- Arctic char
- Bluefish
- Branzino
- Butterfish
- Canned tuna, in water
- Carp
- Catfish
- Caviar
- Clams
- Cod
- Crabmeat, lump
- Crayfish
- Cuttlefish
- Dungeness crab
- Eel
- Fish roe
- Flounder
- Grouper
- Haddock
- Halibut
- Herring
- Lobster
- Mahi mahi
- Monkfish
- Mussels
- Octopus
- Orange roughy
- Oysters
- Perch
- Pike
- Pollock
- Pompano
- Salmon
- Sardines, canned in water or sauce
- Sashimi
- Scallops
- Sea bass
- Sea cucumber
- Sea urchin
- Shrimp
- Smelt
- Smoked haddock
- Smoked salmon
- Smoked sturgeon
- Smoked trout
- Smoked whitefish
- Snails
- Snapper
- Sole
- Squid

Zero Point Drinks

- Water
- Coffee, black (without sugar)
- Coke Zero (all varieties)
- Diet Coke (all varieties)
- Fresca (all varieties)
- Gatorade Zero
- Sparkling Ice Water (all flavors)
- Tea, black
- Vitamin Water Zero

Zero Point Snacks

- Applesauce, unsweetened
- Fruit cup (canned in water pack, no sugar added)
- Fruit cup (fresh)
- Vegetable Sticks
- Yogurt (greek, plain, fat-free, unsweetened)

IMPORTANT NOTICE!!!

We chose to make costs low so it can be accessible to everyone who would love to lose weight. As a result, we didn't include pictures for each recipes.

Please, reach out to us at popoolaadenike805@gmail.com if you would like to receive the pictures for each recipes.

HAPPY COOKING!

Made in United States
Troutdale, OR
03/08/2024

18309298R00046